GASTROESOPHAGEAL REFLUX (GER) COOKBOOK

Navigating a GER-Friendly Kitchen: A Comprehensive Cookbook for Symptom Relief and Culinary Enjoyment

Priscilla J. Schulz

Table of Contents

Introduction

Welcome to the Gastroesophageal Reflux Disease (GERD) Cookbook, your comprehensive guide to cooking and eating delicious meals that won't trigger your GERD symptoms. Embark on a culinary journey filled with flavorful recipes that align with your dietary needs, promoting digestive wellness and overall well-being.

Within this cookbook, you'll discover a wealth of recipes designed to minimize heartburn, regurgitation, and other uncomfortable GERD symptoms. We've carefully curated a collection of dishes that are low in acid-producing ingredients and high in nutrient-rich alternatives, ensuring that every meal is both enjoyable and beneficial for your digestion.

Whether you're craving a satisfying breakfast to start your day, a light lunch to nourish your body, or a comforting dinner to end your evening, our recipes will tantalize your taste buds while keeping your GERD under control. We've included a variety of options to suit different preferences and dietary restrictions, ensuring that everyone can find something they'll love.

As you embark on this culinary adventure, you'll learn how to navigate the world of GERD-friendly cooking with confidence. We'll provide you with essential tips and techniques for selecting ingredients, preparing meals, and storing leftovers to minimize the risk of triggering symptoms.

Along the way, you'll discover a world of flavors and textures that will transform your perception of GERD-friendly cuisine. From refreshing salads and hearty soups to flavorful main courses and delectable desserts, our recipes will prove that eating healthy and managing GERD can go hand in hand.

With this cookbook as your guide, you'll empower yourself to take control of your GERD and enjoy a life filled with delicious and nutritious meals. Embrace the joy of cooking and savor the satisfaction of creating meals that are both tasty and gentle on your digestive system. Let your kitchen become a haven for GERD-friendly culinary creations, and embark on a journey of culinary wellness and delicious living.

CHAPTER ONE

Introduction to Gastroesophageal Reflux Disease (GERD)

The common digestive ailment known as gastroesophageal reflux disease (GERD), or heartburn, is brought on by stomach acid constantly flowing back up into the esophagus, the tube that runs from your mouth to your stomach. This reflux of acid can irritate the lining of the esophagus, leading to a host of painful symptoms, including dry cough, heartburn, and regurgitation of acid.

What Are the Causes

The lower esophageal sphincter (LES), a muscle valve that divides the esophagus from the stomach, is the primary cause of GERD. Stomach acid can reflux into the esophagus when the lower esophageal sphincter (LES) relaxes improperly or at the wrong moment.

Factors that contribute to LES dysfunction and GERD

The disorder known as a hiatal hernia occurs when a portion of the stomach pushes through the diaphragm, the muscle that divides the chest from the abdomen. As a result, the LES may become weaker and more prone to relax.

- Specific foods and drinks: Chocolate, caffeine, alcohol, fatty and spicy foods, and carbonated drinks can all relax the LES and cause reflux.

- Cigarette Use: Smoking has the potential to weaken the LES and raise stomach acid output.

- Growth: Pregnant women are more prone to GERD due to hormonal changes that relax the LES.

- Fatality: Carrying too much weight around the abdomen might compress the stomach and make reflux more likely.

Further variables that could lead to GERD include:

- Specific drugs: Certain drugs, such aspirin, ibuprofen, and some antidepressants, might cause the LES to relax or produce more stomach acid.

- Delayed gastric emptying: A condition where food passes through the stomach more slowly than usual, perhaps increasing the risk of reflux.

- Consuming substantial meals: Large meals have the potential to overburden the LES and increase its propensity to open, which would allow stomach acid to reflux into the esophagus.

- Lying down following a meal: After eating, lying down may facilitate the reflux of stomach acid into the esophagus.

Note: Stress can worsen GERD symptoms by raising the production of stomach acid.

GERD risk factors:

- Age: Adults are more likely than children to have GERD.

- Sex: GERD is more common in men than in women.

- Hereditary: Your chance of having GERD may be raised if you have a family history of the illness.

GERD Prevention:

You can take several measures to avoid developing GERD, such as:

- Retaining an appropriate weight: If you are fat or overweight, losing weight can help to enhance LES function and relieve strain on your abdomen.

- Avoiding meals and drinks that provoke anxiety: Avoid specific foods and drinks if you are aware that they aggravate your GERD symptoms.

- Giving up smoking: Smoking might cause the LES to weaken and produce more stomach acid.

- Consuming fewer meals: A smaller, more frequent meal schedule will help you have less acid in your stomach overall.

- Avoid eating right before bed: Allow your stomach to empty before turning in for the night.

- Elevating the head of your bed: In order to help stop stomach acid from refluxing up into your esophagus while you sleep, raise the head of your bed by 6 to 8 inches.

- Handling stress: It's critical to discover appropriate coping mechanisms for stress because it might exacerbate the symptoms of GERD.

It's critical to visit a physician if you think you may have GERD in order to receive a diagnosis and treatment plan. Your quality of life can be enhanced and consequences can be avoided with early diagnosis and treatment.

Impact of GERD on daily life

Your daily life may be greatly impacted by GERD, which can negatively affect your social, emotional, and physical health.

Physical Impact

- Heartburn: Heartburn, the most prevalent GERD symptom, is a burning feeling in the chest that can be mild to severe. There are specific meals, drinks, and activities that can cause it.

- Recapitulation: Regurgitation, or the sensation of sour or bitter taste in the mouth, is caused by stomach acid pouring back up into the esophagus. Additionally, it may result in a dry cough, hoarseness, and trouble swallowing.

- Heart ache: Chest pain that resembles a heart attack can occasionally be caused by GERD. This may cause needless worry and hospital appointments, and it can be highly concerning.

- Disturbances in sleep: Acid reflux during the night can cause sleep disturbances, exhaustion, and somnolence during the day.

Emotional Effect

- Stress and anxiety: Stress and worry might result from GERD's ongoing discomfort and uncertainty. Individuals who have GERD may be concerned about how their condition may affect their lives, their capacity to manage it, and their symptoms.

- Depression: GERD can have a detrimental effect on one's mood and quality of life, which can result in pessimism and depression.

- Embarrassment in public: GERD symptoms can be awkward and interfere with socializing and enjoyment of hobbies. Those who have GERD may stay away from social events, travel, and dining out of fear of developing symptoms.

Impact on Everyday Activities

- Productivity at work: GERD symptoms can make it difficult to concentrate, maintain focus, and finish activities at work, which can reduce productivity.

- Activities in the body: Exercise and physical activity can be challenging for those with GERD, particularly when it comes to bending or lifting.

- Eating patterns and diet: Food and eating habits might be restricted by GERD since those who have it may abstain from particular meals and drinks that make their symptoms worse.

- Enjoyment of life: GERD can severely affect one's ability to enjoy life in general, which can have an influence on relationships, activities, and general well-being.

Managing GERD's Impact

- Changes in lifestyle: Changing one's lifestyle is frequently the first step in treating GERD. This includes staying away from trigger foods and drinks, keeping a healthy weight, giving up smoking, and controlling stress.

- Prescription: Heartburn reducers and antacids are examples of over-the-counter drugs that can temporarily relieve GERD symptoms. In order to neutralize or lessen the production of stomach acid, prescription drugs may also be recommended.

- Medicine: Surgery might be an option in extreme circumstances in order to reinforce the LES and stop reflux.

Coping with GERD

- Seek assistance: Consult your physician, a therapist, or support groups on GERD's psychological and social effects. You can develop coping mechanisms and feel less alone by talking about your experiences.

- Educate yourself: Gaining knowledge about GERD's causes, triggers, and available treatments will help you take better care of your illness.

- Have patience: GERD management requires patience and work. If you don't notice results right away, don't give up.

- Make self-care a priority: Schedule time for hobbies and relaxation techniques like yoga, meditation, or physical activity.

You can minimize the impact of your GERD on your everyday life and control its symptoms with appropriate management.

Managing GERD with lifestyle modifications and dietary changes

A good way to manage GERD and reduce symptoms while also enhancing general health is to make dietary and lifestyle adjustments. Here's a thorough how-to for implementing these adjustments in your day-to-day activities:

Dietary Adjustments

1. Recognise and Steer Clear of Trigger Foods: To find foods that consistently cause GERD symptoms, keep a meal

journal. Foods high in fat, spice, chocolate, caffeine, alcohol, and carbonated drinks are common offenders.

2. Consume Regular, Smaller Meals: Big meals might put too much strain on the digestive system and raise the risk of reflux. To keep food moving through the stomach consistently, choose to eat smaller, more frequent meals throughout the day.

3. Take Your Time and Chew Carefully: Eat slowly and completely chew your food before swallowing. This lessens the chance of heartburn and helps with digestion.

4. Steer clear of late-night eating: Before lying down, give your stomach enough time to empty. To avoid acid reflux while you sleep, avoid eating for three hours before bed.

5. Raise Your Head While You Sleep: Use blocks or pillows to raise the head of your bed by six to eight inches. This helps prevent acid reflux from the stomach into the esophagus during sleep.

6. Retain a Weight That Is Healthy: Being overweight puts strain on the abdomen and raises the risk of reflux. Maintain a healthy weight range by eating a well-balanced diet and getting frequent exercise.

7. Select Healthful Fats: Choose fats that are better for you, including those in nuts, avocados, and olive oil, rather than trans and saturated fats, which can make GERD symptoms worse.

8. Eat Foods High in Fibre: Fibre can lessen the chance of reflux and aid in digestion regulation. Consume a diet

high in whole grains, fruits, and vegetables that are high in fiber.

9. Restrict Sugar-Coated Drinks: Sugary drinks, such juices and sodas, can exacerbate the symptoms of GERD by increasing the production of acid. Opt instead for unsweetened beverages or water.

10. Take Peppermint Into Account: Natural antispasmodic qualities of peppermint can ease heartburn and relax the digestive system. After meals, think of drinking peppermint tea or sucking on peppermint candies.

Changes in Lifestyle

1. Give Up Smoking: Smoking weakens the LES, increasing the likelihood that it may relax and permit reflux of stomach

acid. Giving up smoking is essential for managing GERD well.

2. Control Tension: GERD symptoms can worsen with stress. To encourage relaxation, try stress-reduction methods like yoga, meditation, or deep breathing exercises.

3. Put on loose-fitting attire: Clothing that is too tight around the abdomen might press on the stomach and raise the possibility of reflux. Choose loose-fitting clothing to facilitate easy digestion.

4. Elevate the Head of Your Bed: Use cushions or blocks to raise the head of your bed by 6 to 8 inches. This helps prevent acid reflux from the stomach into the esophagus during sleep.

5. Refrain from Lying Down Right After Eating: To avoid acid reflux, avoid

reclining or lying down for three hours after eating. To help with digestion, sit up straight or do simple activities.

6. After Meals, Chew Gum: Gum chewing increases saliva production, which can lessen the chance of reflux and assist balance stomach acid.

7. Refrain from Working Out After Eating: Steer clear of intense exercise right after eating as this can exacerbate reflux and raise stomach pressure. A minimum of two hours should pass between meals and physical activity.

8. Maintain a Healthy Sleep Schedule: Try to get between seven and eight hours of good sleep every night. Getting enough sleep lowers the chance of reflux and aids in the regulation of hormones that govern digestion.

Recall that GERD management is a continuous effort. Finding the exact triggers you experience and the dietary and lifestyle adjustments that work best for you may take some time. For individualized advice and assistance, speak with your healthcare professional and exercise patience and consistency.

CHAPTER TWO

GERD-Friendly Cooking Principles

1. Identifying and avoiding trigger foods

The first step in controlling GERD symptoms and enhancing general health is recognising and avoiding trigger foods. This is a thorough guide to helping you identify and stay away from your unique GERD triggers:

1. Record Your Food

Keeping a meal journal is the best method for determining your unique causes for GERD. For a duration of two to four weeks, keep a log of your meals, snacks, and drinks, indicating the time and date of each food item you consume.

2. Take Note of Symptoms

Note any symptoms of gastric reflux disease (GERD), such as heartburn, acid reflux, chest pain, or difficulty swallowing, along with the food you eat. Take note of each symptom's length and intensity.

3. Examine Trends

Once food consumption and symptoms are regularly monitored, examine the trends to find foods or drinks that either regularly precede or coincide with GERD symptoms. These foods could be triggers for you.

4. Get Rid of Possible Triggers

For two to four weeks, cut out the foods that you feel are triggers from your diet. Keep an eye out for any decrease in or removal of your GERD symptoms during this elimination phase.

5. Gradually Reintroduce Foods

Once possible triggers have been eliminated, reintroduce them one at a time while closely monitoring your symptoms. Once a specific meal is again consumed, if symptoms reappear, identify it as a trigger and consistently avoid it.

6. Customized Methodology

Keep in mind that every person has different GERD triggers. Although there are common triggers, it's important to determine your own triggers by thorough observation and removal.

Regular Causes of GERD

- Fatty meals: Certain meals might relax the LES and increase reflux, such as fatty meats, fried foods, whole-fat dairy products, and full-fat desserts.

- Spicy Foods: Spicy condiments, hot sauces, and chili peppers might increase GERD symptoms by irritating the lining of the esophagus.

- Chocolate: Caffeine and cocoa, two ingredients in chocolate, have the ability to relax the LES and cause reflux.

- Coffee: Caffeine is an ingredient in coffee, tea, sodas, and energy beverages. It can increase the production of stomach acid and exacerbate the symptoms of GERD.

- Alcohol: Drinking alcohol can cause reflux episodes by relaxing the LES and producing more stomach acid.

- Carbonated Drinks: Carbonated beverages like sodas and seltzer water have the potential to dilate the stomach and cause acid to rise into the esophagus.

- Foods That Are Acidic: Tomatoes, vinegars, and citrus fruits can all cause reflux by producing more stomach acid.

- Mind: Spearmint and peppermint can relax the LES and exacerbate the symptoms of GERD.

More Advice on Recognising Triggers

- Think About Meal Timing: Check to see whether certain meals or snacks—like late-night or large meals—have a greater effect on symptoms.

- Keep an eye on your stress levels: GERD symptoms may get worse under stress. Observe whether symptoms intensify during times of stress.

- Speak with a Medical Professional: For individualized advice and support, talk to your physician or a qualified dietician about your probable triggers.

Recall that recognising and staying away from trigger foods is a continuous effort. To properly manage your GERD, keep a close eye on your symptoms and adapt as necessary.

2. **Choosing low-fat, lean protein sources**

An important component of a diet that is GERD-friendly is lean protein sources. Protein is a necessary food for sustaining body functioning, growing muscular growth, and encouraging fullness. But controlling the symptoms of GERD requires selecting the correct sources of protein.

Advantages of Lean, Low-Fat Protein

- Decreases Intake of Fat: The Lower Esophageal Sphincter (LES), a valve that keeps stomach acid from refluxing into the esophagus, might relax when fatty meats are consumed. Choosing lean protein sources minimizes the risk of reflux by drastically reducing total fat intake.

- Encourages Simple Digestion: Generally speaking, lean proteins are simpler to digest than fatty meats, which eases the strain on the digestive system and avoids pain.

- Offers Vital Nutrients: Iron, zinc, and B vitamins are among the vital elements found in lean protein sources, without the added fat that may aggravate GERD symptoms.

Instances of Lean, Low-Fat Protein Sources

- Vegetables: Turkey and skinless chicken are great, low-fat, easily digested sources of lean protein. They can be baked, grilled, or poached, among other preparation methods.

- A fish: Omega-3 fatty acids are abundant in fish, especially oily fish like mackerel, tuna, and salmon. These fatty acids have anti-inflammatory qualities and may help lessen the symptoms of GERD. Bake, poach, or grill fish to reduce the amount of fat added.

- Tofu: A flexible protein source derived from soy that is low in fat and cholesterol is tofu. It takes well to a variety of cooking techniques, including baking, grilling, and stir-frying. It also absorbs the flavors of sauces and spices.

- Verdures: Peas, beans, and lentils are great plant-based protein sources that are low in fat and high in fiber. They go well with salads, dips, stews, and soups.

- Eggs: Egg holes offer more nutrients, whereas egg whites are a low-fat, high-protein source. If you want a lower-fat option, go with egg whites.

Guides for Selecting Sources of Lean Protein

- Examine food labels: When selecting packaged protein sources, be sure to take into account the amount of fat per serving. Select products that are lower in fat and saturated fat.

- Trim Visible Fat: To lower total fat content, trim visible fat and skin from meats prior to cooking.

- Cooking Methods: Select cooking techniques like grilling, baking, broiling, or poaching that call for the least amount of oil or fat.

- Portion Control: Watch how much you eat. Even with lean protein sources, overindulging can strain the digestive tract and raise the risk of reflux.

Low-fat protein sources in your diet are crucial for GERD symptom management and general health maintenance. You may have healthy meals without making your GERD worse by selecting lean protein options and cooking them properly.

3.Incorporating low-acid fruits and vegetables

Rich in vitamins, minerals, fiber, and antioxidants, fruits and vegetables are vital parts of a balanced diet. On the other hand, choosing low-acid fruits and vegetables is essential for people with GERD in order to reduce possible triggers and support overall digestive health.

Advantages of Fruits and Vegetables Low in Acid

- Decreased Acid Reflux: Fruits and vegetables with low acid content have less of an effect on the creation of stomach acid, which lowers the risk of heartburn and reflux episodes.

- High Fiber Content: These foods are high in fiber, which lowers the risk of overeating and reflux by promoting fullness, slowing down the passage of food through the digestive tract, and regulating digestion.

- Nutrient-Dense: Packed with vital nutrients, low-acid fruits and vegetables promote general health and offer antioxidants that may help fend against chronic illnesses.

Instances of Fruits and Vegetables with Low Acidity

- Watermelons:Cantaloupe, honeydew melons, and watermelon are all great options because of their low acidity and high water content.

- Bananas: In addition to being naturally low in acid, bananas are a significant source of potassium.

- Apples: Apples are high in fiber and antioxidants and have a comparatively low acid content, especially the Granny Smith and Red Delicious varieties.

- Apples: Pears' low acidity and high fiber content make them generally well-tolerated by GERD sufferers.

- Verdant Produce: Celery, lettuce, cauliflower, broccoli, cucumbers, celery and zucchini are low-acid vegetables that are gentle on the stomach.

- Vegetables with Roots: Due to their comparatively low acid content, starchy vegetables like sweet potatoes, carrots, and parsnips make good choices.

Guides for Including Fruits and Vegetables with Low Acidity

- Type: To optimize nutritional intake and appreciate a range of flavors and textures, try to eat a variety of low-acid fruits and vegetables.

- Preparation Techniques: Use cooking techniques like steaming, roasting, or grilling to maximize the preservation of nutrients and reduce the addition of fat.

- Control of Points: Pay attention to portion proportions to prevent overindulging and possible gastrointestinal distress.

- Time of Consumption: Steer clear of consuming a lot of fruits and vegetables right before bed, as this can raise your risk of experiencing reflux while you sleep.

Fruits and vegetables with low acidity are important parts of a diet that is GERD-friendly. These nutrient-dense foods can help you maintain digestive health, control the symptoms of GERD, and eat a well-balanced, healthful diet.

4. Selecting healthy fats and cooking methods

Your general health and well-being depend on including healthy fats in your diet. To reduce possible triggers and enhance digestive comfort, choosing the appropriate fats is essential for those with GERD.

Healthy Fats' Benefits

- Decrease Arthritis: The anti-inflammatory qualities of healthy fats, especially polyunsaturated and monounsaturated fats, may help lessen the symptoms of GERD.

- Encourage the Absorption of Nutrients: The absorption of fat-soluble vitamins, including A, D, E, and K, is facilitated by healthy fats.

- Encourage Heart Health: In order to improve heart health, healthy fats can help boost HDL (good) cholesterol and decrease LDL (bad) cholesterol.

Instances of Nutritious Fats

- Olive Oil: Olive oil is a great option for GERD because it's high in antioxidants and monounsaturated fats.

- Oil of Avocado: Avocado oil is a good source of monounsaturated fats and has a high smoke point.

- Nut Oils: Almond, hazelnut, and walnut oils are excellent providers of mono- and polyunsaturated fats.

- Fats from Nuts and Seeds: Nuts and seeds, including flaxseeds, chia seeds, walnuts, and almonds, offer fiber and healthy fats.

GERD Cooking Techniques

Cooking techniques have a big impact on how healthy your meals are overall and how much fat they contain. By using

GERD-friendly cooking methods, you can reduce possible triggers and encourage comfort in the digestive system. Suggested Cooking Techniques

- Heating up: Steaming is a low-fat cooking technique that retains moisture and nutrients. It works best with fish, veggies, and lean proteins.

- Location: Food is poached by simmering it in a liquid (usually broth or water) without using any heat. For delicate meals like fish, poultry, and veggies, this approach works well.

- Creaming: Baking is the process of cooking food in an oven with dry heat. It's an adaptable technique that works well with a variety of foods, such as baked items, seafood, veggies, and lean meats.

- Simmering: When food is broiled, it is cooked over high heat in a grill or grill, producing a crispy outside and a juicy inside. It goes well with fish, meats, and veggies.

- Chewing Food that has been grilling is cooked over direct fire, which gives it a smoky flavor and charred edges. Because it uses less oil than pan-frying, it's a healthier option.

Guides for Choosing Nutritious Fats and Cooking Techniques

- Limit Added Fats: To reduce the total fat level of your meals, use less added fats such butter, margarine, and shortening.

- Moderate Use of Oil: Use healthy oils sparingly because, when taken in excess, even good fats can aggravate reflux.

- Season with Herbs and Spices: Rather than depending solely on thick sauces or butter, amp up flavor with herbs and spices.

- Avoid Deep-Frying: Deep-frying increases calories and fat content while exacerbating symptoms of GERD.

- Remove Extra Fat: To lower fat intake, remove extra fat from meats and poultry after cooking.

Choosing healthy fats and cooking techniques are crucial for controlling GERD symptoms and enhancing general health. You can have tasty and fulfilling meals without making your

GERD worse by implementing these strategies into your cooking practice.

5. **Preparing meals that are easy to digest**

Eating foods that are easy on the digestive tract is important because GERD can affect digestion severely. Here are some broad pointers for choosing foods that are simple to digest:

- Sources of low-fat protein: Choose lean protein sources such as beans, fish, tofu, eggs, and skinless chicken. These proteins digest more readily and are less prone to produce symptoms of reflux.

- Vegetables and fruits with low acidity: Add a range of low-acid fruits and vegetables, including carrots, sweet potatoes, broccoli, cauliflower, apples, pears, and melons. These foods encourage comfort in the digestive system and are less prone to irritate the esophagus.

- Whole grains: Opt for whole grains rather than refined ones since they include fiber, which slows down food transit through the digestive tract and helps with digestion.

- Properly prepared food: Cook food to the right temperature to break down the fibers and facilitate digestion. Steer clear of raw meals since they could be harder to digest.

Preparation Techniques for Simple Digestion

Certain cooking techniques, which break down fibers and soften textures, can facilitate simpler digestion. The following are some suggested cooking techniques:

- Heating up: For vegetables, lean proteins, and fish, steaming is the best method since it retains moisture and nutrients without adding fat.

- Location: Food is poached by cooking it in a liquid (usually broth or water) without using direct heat, which is gentler on the stomach.

- Creaming: Baking is the process of cooking food in an oven using dry heat, producing foods that are soft and simple to digest.

- Chewing: For lean meats, fish, and vegetables, grilling over direct fire provides flavor and sear without adding extra fat.

Introductory Meal Samples

Easy-to-digest meal ideas to include in your GERD-friendly diet include the following:

- Breakfast

    - Berries and nuts added to muesli

    - Whole-wheat bread with scrambled eggs

    - Fruit and granola paired with yogurt parfait

- Lunch:

- A salad of grilled chicken, mixed greens, with mild vinaigrette

- Whole-grain bread paired with lentil soup

- Roasted vegetable and salmon

- Supper:

    - Baked cod over brown rice and steamed veggies

    - Brown rice with turkey chili

    - Stir-fried veggies with lean protein or tofu

A Guide to Cooking Simple-to-Digest Foods

- Avoid large meals: To ease the strain on your digestive system, choose smaller, more frequent meals.

- Chew everything well and slowly: Food is broken down into smaller, more digestible pieces when it is chewed properly.

- Avoid eating late at night: Give yourself enough time to finish eating before turning in to sleep to avoid reflux.

- Remain hydrated: To help with digestion and avoid constipation, sip lots of water throughout the day.

- Control your stress: GERD symptoms may get worse under stress. Use stress-reduction methods such as yoga, meditation, or physical activity.

Recall that every GERD patient may have unique triggers and sensitivities. See a trained dietitian or your physician for individualized advice on choosing and preparing meals and foods that are easy to digest.

CHAPTER THREE

Breakfast Recipes for a GERD-Friendly Start

A healthy and adaptable breakfast choice, muesli is also a good fit for those who have GERD. It's a mild and filling option for the beginning of the day because of its high fiber content, moderate acidity, and capacity to absorb stomach acid.

Oatmeal's Benefits for GERD

- High Density: Soluble fiber, found in abundance in muesli, facilitates digestion, controls blood sugar, and increases feelings of fullness. By slowing down the passage of food through the digestive system, fiber lowers the chance of reflux episodes.

- Low Acidity: Because muesli has a low acidity by nature, it is less prone to irritate the esophagus and cause heartburn.

- Absorption of Stomach Acid: Because muesli may absorb stomach acid, it can neutralize excess acid and lessen the symptoms of reflux.

Including Nuts and Berries

Oatmeal's flavor and nutritional content are further improved by adding nuts and berries, all while keeping it GERD-friendly.

- Berries: Strawberries, raspberries, and blueberries are berries that are high in antioxidants and low in acid. They enhance oatmeal's sweetness, flavor, and nutritional value without making GERD symptoms worse.

- Nuts: Nuts include minerals, fiber, protein, and healthy fats. Some examples of nuts are pecans, walnuts, and almonds. They can help keep you feeling full until noon and offer a delicious crunch.

Gerd-Friendly Muesli Preparation

Use these tips to make sure your muesli is GERD-friendly:

- Select Rolled Oats: Choose rolled oats over steel-cut or quick oats since they cook to a creamier texture and contain more fiber.

- Steer clear of added sugars: Avoid pre-flavored muesli or muesli packs that have been sweetened. Alternatively, you can naturally sweeten your muesli by adding cinnamon, honey or berries.

- Reduce Milk or Cream: To reduce fat content, use plant-based milk substitutes or low-fat or non-fat milk. Steer clear of whole milk and heavy cream since these can exacerbate GERD symptoms.

Guides for Snacking on Muesli with Nuts and Berries

- Properly Prepare Muesli: To make sure your muesli is thoroughly cooked and easily digested, follow the cooking instructions on the package.

- Let Muesli Cool: To keep the berries and nuts from disintegrating and losing their texture, let the muesli cool somewhat before adding them.

- Tailor to Taste: Change the quantity of nuts and berries to your preferred level. For variation, try blending and matching other kinds of berries and nuts.

A wholesome, filling, and GERD-friendly breakfast choice that can help control symptoms and support digestive health is muesli with berries and almonds. These easy pointers and recommendations can help you enjoy this filling lunch without sacrificing your comfort.

1. Scrambled eggs with spinach and low-fat cheese

A traditional breakfast staple that is easily modified to fit into a GERD-friendly diet is scrambled eggs. You can make a filling and healthy dinner that is easy on the stomach by adding spinach and low-fat cheese.

Effects of Low-Fat Cheese and Spinach on Scrambled Eggs

- Low Protein: Because they include all nine of the essential amino acids, eggs are a complete protein supply. Easy to digest and less likely to aggravate reflux symptoms is lean protein.

- High in Fiber Spinach: Soluble fiber, found in spinach, slows down food transit through the digestive tract, aids in digestion, and increases feelings of fullness. Reflux episodes may be less common with the help of fiber.

- Low-Fat Cheese: Low-fat cheese offers calcium, vitamin D, and protein without adding extra fat, which can exacerbate GERD symptoms. Select reduced-fat or fat-free options like feta, mozzarella, or Swiss cheese.

How to Make GERD-Friendly Scrambled Eggs with Low-Fat Cheese and Spinach

Use these tips to make sure your scrambled eggs are GERD-friendly:

- Use Non-Stick Pan: To reduce the quantity of oil used for cooking, use a non-stick pan.

Preparation Technique: To keep the eggs from sticking and burning, cook them gently, using low heat and frequent turning.

- Avoid Adding Fat: Keep your pan free of fats such as butter, margarine, or other substances.

- Incorporate Spinach: In the final few minutes of cooking, stir in the chopped spinach to the scrambled eggs. In addition to delivering vitamins, minerals, and fiber, spinach wilts quickly.

- Add Low-Fat Cheese: After the scrambled eggs are cooked, sprinkle low-fat or fat-free cheese on top.

Suggested Uses for Low-Fat Cheese and Spinach in Scrambled Eggs

- Season to Taste: Add a dash of pepper, salt, or herbs and spices like garlic powder, thyme, or oregano to enhance the flavor.

- Combine Whole Grains with: For an extra fiber boost, serve your scrambled eggs with whole-grain crackers or whole-wheat bread.

- Think About Veggies: For added taste and benefits, add additional veggies, such as sliced onions, mushrooms, or bell peppers.

You may personalize this adaptable, healthy, and GERD-friendly breakfast choice, which consists of scrambled eggs with spinach and low-fat cheese. These easy pointers and recommendations will help you enjoy this filling supper without sacrificing the comfort of your digestive system.

2. Yogurt parfait with granola and fruit

Yogurt parfaits are a simple, quick, and adaptable breakfast choice that work well with a GERD-friendly diet. Your digestive system won't suffer from this filling and healthy lunch if you choose low-fat yogurt, add fiber-rich granola, and include berries and other low-acid fruits.

Yoghurt Parfait Benefits for GERD with Granola and Fruit

- Yogurt with Low Fat: Yogurt that is low in fat provides calcium and protein without adding extra fat, which can worsen the symptoms of GERD. Select low-fat plain yogurt instead of flavored or sweetened variants, which could have artificial components and added sugars.

- Granola Rich in Fiber: Granola has fiber, which slows food down its passage through the digestive system, aids in digestion regulation, and increases feelings of fullness. Make your own granola or go for a low-fat, low-sugar brand from the supermarket.

- Fats Low in Acid: Apples, melons, bananas, and berries are among the low-acid fruits that are less prone to irritate the esophagus and cause heartburn. Steer clear of citrus fruits and tomatoes because their acidity might exacerbate the symptoms of GERD.

3. Creating a Yoghurt Parfait with Granola and Fruit That Is GERD-Friendly

Use these tips to make sure your yogurt parfait is GERD-friendly:

- Select Low-Fat Plain Yoghurt: Choose plain, low-fat yogurt that hasn't had any artificial flavors or extra sweeteners. You can add some cinnamon or a honey drizzle to organically sweeten it.

- Control of Points: Take care not to use too much granola as this could add extra fat and calories. Limit each parfait to a ¼ to ½ cup amount.

- Components for Layers: Arrange the fruit, granola, and yogurt in a parfait jar or glass. This keeps the granola from getting too wet and gives you control over how much of each ingredient you use.

- Place fresh fruits on top: Pick low-acid fruits like melons, bananas, and apples, or berries like blueberries, raspberries, and strawberries.

Suggested Uses for Yoghurt Parfait with Fruit and Granola

- Relax Later: Place the parfait in the fridge for at least 30 minutes or overnight if you'd like it cooler.

- Add Extra Crunch: To add even more protein and healthy fats to your parfait, sprinkle chopped nuts, like walnuts or almonds, over top.

- Test Flavours Differently: To discover your favorite flavor combinations, experiment with different combinations of granola and fruits.

A customizable yogurt parfait with fruit and granola is a GERD-friendly, healthful, and refreshing breakfast choice. You can savor this tasty supper without jeopardizing your digestive comfort by following these easy pointers.

4. Smoothies made with low-acid fruits, yogurt, and spinach

A tasty and easy method to add important nutrients to your diet is with smoothies. Low-acid fruits, yogurt, and spinach are good choices for smoothie components to help manage symptoms and support digestive comfort for those who suffer with GERD.

Smoothie Benefits for GERD

- Easy to Digest: Smoothies offer nutrients in a liquid form, which facilitates easy digestion and reduces GERD sufferers' discomfort.

- High Fiber Content: By promoting fullness and slowing down the passage of food through the digestive tract, spinach and other high-fiber foods can help control digestion and lower the risk of overeating and reflux.

- High in Nutrients: Low-acid fruits, yogurt, and spinach may all provide a plethora of vitamins, minerals, and antioxidants to smoothies.

Selecting Fruits Low in Acid for Smoothies

Choose low-acid fruit types for your GERD-friendly smoothies to reduce the possibility of causing reflux symptoms. Suitable options consist of:

- Watermelons: Cantaloupe, honeydew melons, and watermelons are naturally low in acid and high in water content.

- Bananas: Bananas are high in potassium and low in acid.

- Apples: Apples are high in fiber and relatively low in acid, especially the Granny Smith and Red Delicious kinds.

- Apples: Pears' low acidity and high fiber content make them generally well-tolerated by GERD sufferers.

Sweetheart Yogurt

Select non-fat or low-fat yogurt to cut down on fat consumption and lessen the chance of reflux triggers. It is better to stick to plain yogurt since flavored or sweetened variants could have artificial components and extra sugars.

Spinach in Drinks

Soluble fiber, which improves digestion and lowers the risk of reflux episodes, is abundant in spinach. Its subtle flavor goes well in smoothies with different fruits and yogurt.

Guides for Making Smoothies That Are GERD-Friendly

- Make use of a blender: To puree spinach and other ingredients into a smooth, palatable consistency, a strong blender is necessary.

- Add Liquids Gradually: Add a little amount of liquid (water, low-fat milk, or plant-based milk substitutes) at first, then progressively add more until the desired consistency is reached.

- Avoid Sweeteners: Artificial sweeteners and excessive honey should be avoided since they might exacerbate GERD symptoms by increasing acid production.

- Eat Smoothies Right Away: Smoothies should be consumed right away to avoid vitamin oxidation and possible fermentation.

Example Recipes for GERD-Friendly Smoothies

Here are some smoothie recipe examples that are easy on the digestive tract and appropriate for those with GERD:

Spinach and Melon Smoothie:

Components:

- One cup of cubed cantaloupe or watermelon

- A quarter cup of frozen berries (raspberries, blueberries, and strawberries)

- ½ cup of low-fat plain yogurt

- Half a cup of spinach

- As needed, water or low-fat milk

Guidelines:

1. Fill a blender with all the ingredients; process until smooth.

2. If necessary, adjust consistency with more water or reduced-fat milk.

Smoothie with Banana and Spinach:

Components:

- One mature banana

- ½ cup of low-fat plain yogurt

- Half a cup of spinach

- As needed, water or low-fat milk

- An optional pinch of cinnamon

Guidelines:

1. Fill a blender with all the ingredients; process until smooth.

2. If necessary, adjust consistency with more water or reduced-fat milk.

3. For added taste and digestive benefits, sprinkle with a little cinnamon.

Smoothie with Pears and Spinach:

Components:

- One medium-sized pear, cut and cored

- ½ cup of low-fat plain yogurt

- Half a cup of spinach

- As needed, water or low-fat milk

Guidelines:

1. Fill a blender with all the ingredients; process until smooth.

2. If necessary, adjust consistency with more water or reduced-fat milk.

Smoothies with spinach, yogurt, and low-acid fruits are a wholesome and practical approach to improve your general health and control GERD symptoms. Smoothies are tasty and refreshing, and you may enjoy them without sacrificing the comfort of your digestive system by following these easy suggestions and rules.

5. Whole-wheat pancakes with fruit topping

Pancakes made from whole wheat are a filling and healthy breakfast choice that are readily modified to fit within a GERD-friendly diet. You may make a filling dinner that is easy on your stomach by starting with whole-wheat flour, adding low-fat milk or plant-based milk substitutes, and finishing with berries and other low-acid fruits.

Wellness Advantages of Whole-Wheat Pancakes with Fruit Syrup

- Flour Made from Whole Wheat: Rich in dietary fiber, whole-wheat flour facilitates satiety, aids in digestion, and helps control blood sugar levels. By slowing down the passage of food through the digestive system, fiber helps lower the likelihood of reflux episodes.

- Plant-Based Milk Alternatives or Low-Fat Milk: To cut down on fat and lessen the chance of reflux triggers, choose low-fat milk or unsweetened plant-based milk substitutes.

- Low-Acid Fruits: Low-acid fruits like melons, bananas, and apples, as well as berries like blueberries, raspberries, and strawberries, are less prone to irritate the esophagus and cause heartburn.

How to Make Whole-Wheat Pancakes That Are GERD-Friendly

Use these tips to make sure your whole-wheat pancakes are GERD-friendly:

- Select whole-wheat flour. To improve the overall nutrient profile and boost fiber content, use whole-wheat flour rather than refined flour.

- Maximum Fat: Steer clear of adding margarine or butter to the batter. To reduce the amount of extra fat required for cooking, use a non-stick pan.

- Control Oil Usage: To keep the pancakes from sticking to the pan, lightly spray the pan with cooking spray or use a small amount of oil.

- Preparation Technique: To avoid burning and to ensure that they cook evenly throughout, cook the pancakes over low to medium heat.

Adding Fruit As a Topping

Top your pancakes with low-acid fruits for a little sweetness and nutritional value. Here are some pointers:

- New Fruits: For the topping, pick ripe, fresh berries or other low-acid fruits.

- Avoid Added Sugars: Syrups, jams, and other sugary toppings should be avoided since they may exacerbate the symptoms of GERD.

- Fruit Variety: To discover your favorite flavor combinations, try combining various berries and other fruits in different combinations.

Suggested Servings

For a well-rounded and filling breakfast, serve your whole-wheat pancakes with a fruit topping and a side of protein, like a poached egg or a dollop of low-fat Greek yogurt.

You can personalize these whole-wheat pancakes with fruit topping to make a satisfying, high-fiber, and GERD-friendly morning choice. You can enjoy this tasty and nutritious dinner without jeopardizing your digestive comfort by following these easy instructions and advice.

CHAPTER FOUR

Lunchtime Delights that Won't Upset Your Stomach

1. Salads with grilled chicken or fish, low-acid fruits, and leafy greens

Salads offer a nutrient-dense, light, and refreshing lunch choice that is easily adapted to a diet favorable for those with GERD. Low-acid fruits, leafy greens, and grilled chicken or fish can all be combined to provide a filling, tasty lunch that is easy on the stomach.

Salads' Benefits for GERD

- Simple to Process: The nutrients in salads are typically simple to digest, which eases the strain on the digestive system.

- Low Fat Content: Lean protein, such as that found in grilled chicken or fish, does not contain added fat, which can worsen the symptoms of GERD.

- Leafy Greens Rich in Fibre: Leafy greens, such romaine lettuce, spinach, and kale, are great providers of dietary fiber that facilitates satiety, aids in digestion, and helps control blood sugar levels. By slowing down the passage of food through the digestive system, fiber helps lower the likelihood of reflux episodes.

- Low-Acid Fruits: Low-acid fruits like melons, bananas, and apples, as well as berries like blueberries, raspberries, and strawberries, are less prone to irritate the esophagus and cause heartburn.

Selecting Grilled Species for Salads

Choose grilled chicken or fish for your protein source in a salad to make it GERD-friendly. These options for lean protein are easy to digest and low in fat.

- Charbroiled Chicken: To make sure the skinless chicken breast or thigh is thoroughly cooked and safe to eat, broil it until the internal temperature reaches 165°F (74°C).

- Grilled Fish: Opt for mild, low-fat fish choices, including tilapia, salmon, or cod. For the best doneness, grill the salmon until the internal temperature reaches 145°F, or 63°C.

Adding Fruits with Low Acidity

Toss in some low-acid fruits to give your salad a little sweetness and great nutrition.

- New Fruits: For the salad, choose ripe, fresh berries or other low-acid fruits.

- Fruit Variety: To discover your favorite flavor combinations, try combining various berries and other fruits in different combinations.

Choosing Verdant Greens

To increase vitamin intake and add texture to your salad, use a variety of leafy greens.

- Verdant: A great source of fiber, vitamins, and minerals is spinach. Its subtle flavor complements the other elements in salads perfectly.

- Kale: Kale is a leafy green that is high in nutrients and has a hint of pepper. It offers antioxidants, vitamins, and fiber.

- Lettuce: Romaine A crisp and pleasant lettuce kind that gives a neutral flavor to salads is romaine.

More Advice for Making Salads That Are GERD-Friendly

- Steer clear of creamy dressings: Rather than creamy sauces that could have extra sugars and fats, choose for lighter dressings like balsamic vinegar or vinaigrette.

- Herbs and Spices for the Season: Use herbs and spices like oregano, basil, thyme, or a dash of black pepper to enhance the flavor of your salad.

- Moderate Oil Usage: To add taste and good fats without going overboard, lightly sprinkle on some avocado or olive oil.

- Steer clear of acidic ingredients: Avoid foods like pickles, tomatoes, and citrus fruits as they might cause reflux symptoms due to their acidic nature.

Model Salad Mixtures

Here are some flavor-filled and GERD-friendly sample salad combinations:

- Grilled Spinach and Berry Chicken Salad: Add grilled chicken breast, spinach, and a vinaigrette dressing to a bowl.

Grilled Kale and Apple Salad with Salmon: Combine diced apples, chopped kale, grilled salmon, and balsamic vinaigrette dressing.

- Grilled Shrimp Salad with Romaine Lettuce and Avocado: Combine romaine lettuce, grilled shrimp, avocado slices and a mild vinaigrette dressing.

A healthy, GERD-friendly lunch option is a salad with grilled chicken or fish, leafy greens, and low-acid fruits. These easy pointers and recommendations will help you enjoy tasty and filling salads without sacrificing the comfort of your digestive system.

2. Soups made with low-acid vegetables and lean protein

Soups are a satisfying, hydrating, and nutrient-dense meal option that are readily incorporated into a diet that is GERD-friendly. You may make a pleasant and tasty soup that is easy on your digestive system by choosing low-acid veggies, lean protein sources, and mild cooking techniques.

Soups' Benefits for GERD

- Simple to Process: Because of their liquid form, soups are often easy on the digestive system to process.

- Surfactant: Soups can help lessen the symptoms of acid reflux and offer vital hydration, which is important for general health.

- High Fiber Content: Carrots, celery, and potatoes are examples of low-acid vegetables that are high in fiber. Fiber slows down food transit through the digestive tract, aids in digestion, and increases feelings of fullness. Reflux episodes may be less common with the help of fiber.

- Lean Protein: Foods high in lean protein, including fish, poultry, or beans, supply important amino acids without adding extra fat, which can exacerbate the symptoms of GERD.

Selecting Low-Acid Soup Vegetables

Choose low-acid vegetables for your GERD-friendly soups to reduce the likelihood of producing reflux symptoms. Suitable options consist of:

- Veggies: Beta-carotene, fiber, and vitamins are all present in good amounts in carrots. They give soups a hint of sweetness and have a moderate flavor.

- Celery: Celery is a vegetable high in fiber, potassium, and vitamin K that is low in calories. It gives soups crispness and tastes refreshing.

- Care: Potassium and fiber are abundant in potatoes. Select starchy potato cultivars such as russets or white potatoes. Don't eat acidic potatoes, such as tomatoes.

Choosing Sources of Lean Protein

Add lean protein sources to your GERD-friendly soups to help satisfy your hunger and supply necessary amino acids.

- A chicken Choose skinless chicken breasts or thighs as they are easier to digest and have less fat. For the soup, you can shred or cube the chicken after grilling, baking, or poaching it.

- A fish Opt for mild, low-fat fish types like tilapia, salmon, or cod. Fish can be baked, grilled, or poached and then flaked into the soup.

- Beans: Fiber and protein are also found in beans, making them a great plant-based protein source. Go for beans that are simple to digest, including black beans, chickpeas, or lentils.

Preparing Soups That Are GERD-Friendly

To retain nutrients and reduce the production of unpleasant chemicals, heat food gently.

- Inserting: Flavors can develop as components are simmered over low heat without overcooking the protein or veggies.

- Location: Food is poached by simmering it in a liquid (usually broth or water) without using any heat. Fish and poultry are examples of delicate ingredients that work well with this moderate technique.

- Heating up: Vegetables can be kept nutrient- and moisture-rich without overcooking by steaming. Vegetables can be steamed in the soup pot itself or with the use of an additional steamer basket.

Guides for Making Soups That Are GERD-Friendly

- Steer clear of acidic ingredients: Acidic foods and substances (such as tomatoes, citrus fruits, and pickles) should be avoided as they may aggravate reflux symptoms.

- Reduce Fat: When cooking protein or sautéing veggies, use as little oil or fat as possible. To lessen the need for additional fat, you can also use a nonstick pan.

- Herbs and Spices for the Season: Use herbs and spices like oregano, basil, thyme, or a dash of black pepper to enhance the flavor of your soup. Steer clear of strong spices or condiments that could aggravate the esophagus.

- Adjust Consistency: Change the soup's consistency by adding or removing broth or water. For a smoother texture, you can alternatively purée the soup using an immersion blender.

Example Recipes for Soup

A few flavorful and GERD-friendly sample soup recipes are shown below:

- Vegetable Soup with Chicken: Add the cooked chicken, celery, carrots, potatoes, and a thin broth to the mixture. Simmer the veggies until they are soft.

- Spinach Lentil Soup: Combine lentils with a vegetable broth, spinach, carrots, and onions.

Simmer until spinach is wilted and lentils are tender.

- Soup with Salmon and Potatoes: Simmer potatoes, carrots, onions, and salmon filets in a mild broth. Simmer until the fish is cooked through and the veggies are soft.

Low-acid vegetable and lean protein soups are a flexible, wholesome, and GERD-friendly supper choice. These easy pointers and recommendations will help you make tasty soups that satisfy your cravings without sacrificing the comfort of your digestive system.

3. **Whole-wheat sandwiches with lean protein, low-acid vegetables, and low-fat spreads**

Sandwiches made with whole wheat provide a quick, easy, and adaptable dinner alternative that is suitable for GERD sufferers. You can make a filling, healthy sandwich that is easy on your stomach by selecting whole-wheat bread, adding lean protein sources, low-acid veggies, and utilizing low-fat spreads.

Whole-wheat sandwich Benefits for GERD

- Bread Made Whole Wheat: Fibre from whole-wheat bread facilitates satiety, aids in digestion, and helps control blood sugar levels. By slowing down the passage of food through the digestive system, fiber helps lower the likelihood of reflux episodes.

- Lean Protein: Proteins that are low in fat, including skinless chicken or fish, supply vital amino acids without exacerbating the symptoms of GERD.

- Vegetables Low in Acid: Including vegetables with low acidity, such lettuce, cucumbers, and bell peppers, gives you vitamins, minerals, and fiber without making your reflux worse.

- Fat-Free Spreads: Avoid high-fat spreads like butter or full-fat mayonnaise, which can exacerbate the symptoms of GERD. Instead, use low-fat spreads like hummus, avocado spread, or light mayonnaise.

Selection of Whole-Wheat Bread

Choose whole-wheat breads that are low in refined carbs and high in fiber for your GERD-friendly sandwiches.

- Complete-Wheat Types: To be sure the bread is mostly produced with whole-wheat flour, look for labels that say "whole-wheat" or "100% whole-wheat."

- Content of Fiber: Look up the bread's fiber content on the label. Choose bread that provides three grams or more of fiber per serving.

- Examine the Ingredient List: Steer clear of bread that has artificial chemicals, extra sugars, or preservatives.

Choosing Sources of Lean Protein

Add lean protein sources to your GERD-friendly sandwiches to help satisfy your appetite and supply vital amino acids.

- Chicken Without Skin: Choose skinless chicken breasts or thighs as they are easier to digest and have less fat. The chicken can be poached, baked, or grilled before being thinly sliced for the sandwich.

- A fish: Opt for mild, low-fat fish types like tilapia, salmon, or cod. Fish can be baked, grilled, or poached and then flaked into the sandwich.

- Eggs: For a sandwich, eggs can be fried in a light coating, scrambled, or hard-boiled. They are a versatile protein choice.

Using Vegetables Low in Acid

To enhance the taste and nutritional value of your sandwiches, incorporate an assortment of low-acid veggies.

- Cabbage: Lettuce gives the sandwich fiber, vitamins, and minerals without making it more acidic. Select types such as arugula, spinach, or romaine lettuce.

- Cucumbers: Low in calories and acidity, cucumbers are a pleasant and hydrating vegetable. Thinly slice them for the sandwich.

- Spicy Bell Peppers: Bell peppers are an excellent source of antioxidants and vitamin C. To get a range of colors and flavors, choose for bell peppers that are red, green, or yellow.

Selecting Spreads Low in Fat

To cut down on fat content and lower the chance of reflux triggers, choose low-fat spreads rather than high-fat spreads.

- Hummus: A spread made from chickpeas, hummus is rich in protein, fiber, and good fats. It gives sandwiches a savory flavor and creamy texture.

- Spread of Avocado: Avocado spread is a great way to get vitamins, fiber, and good fats. To make avocados spreadable, mash and season them.

- Light Mayonnaise: To lower the fat level, use low-fat or light mayonnaise rather than regular mayonnaise.

Guides for Making Sandwiches That Are GERD-Friendly

- Bread Toasting: Toasting the bread can help it become less moist and simpler to break down.

- Portion Control: To prevent overindulging and possible reflux issues, use modest amounts of spreads and protein.

- Steer clear of acidic ingredients: Acidic foods and substances (such as tomatoes, citrus fruits, and pickles) should be avoided as they may aggravate reflux symptoms.

- Herbs and Spices for the Season: Use herbs and spices like oregano, basil, thyme, or a dash of black pepper to enhance the flavor of your sandwich. Steer clear of strong spices or condiments that could aggravate the esophagus.

Instance Sandwich Orders

These are a few GERD-friendly, flavor-packed sample sandwich combinations:

Grilled Chicken Sandwich with Cucumber and Hummus: Top toasted whole-wheat toast with grilled chicken breast, hummus, sliced cucumbers, and lettuce.

4. Leftovers from the previous night's dinner

Although they are frequently disregarded as a meal option, leftovers may be a fantastic way to save time, cut down on food waste, and have a satisfying and wholesome meal. Making use of last night's meal leftovers has a number of benefits:

- Length: Having leftovers helps cut down on food waste, which is a big environmental problem. You may conserve resources and lessen the environmental effect of food production by eating leftovers, which will reduce the quantity of food that ends up in landfills.

- Affordability: When you're pressed for time or energy, leftovers are a convenient and speedy dinner choice. For an easy dinner, just reheat or repurpose the leftovers.

- Selection: You can eat a different meal than your dinner if you have leftovers. Use your imagination to create new meals out of leftovers or toss them into salads, stir-fries, or soups.

- **Economic Viability:** Because leftovers make use of food that has already been bought, they help you stretch your grocery budget. This might be very helpful for people or families that are on a limited budget.

Guides for Making the Most of Leftovers

Use these pointers to get the most out of leftovers:

- **Appropriate Storage:** To preserve freshness and avoid spoiling, store leftovers right away in airtight containers or securely wrapped in plastic wrap. After cooking, store leftovers in the refrigerator or freeze them.

- **Heating Techniques:** To avoid overcooking and maintain

nutrients, use mild reheating techniques like steaming, low-power microwaving, or warming in a skillet over low heat.

- Using Leftovers Again: Utilize leftovers creatively by incorporating them into new meals. Grilled chicken shreds can be used as a pizza topping or added to salads. Use leftover veggies to make a filling stir-fry or soup.

- Preparation in Advance: Arrange things in advance to maximize leftovers. When preparing meals, cook additional portions, paying special attention to foods that reheat nicely.

Model Remainder Modifications

Here are some suggestions for creating new meals with leftovers:

- Remaining Roast Chicken: Use the chicken shreds in wraps, salads, and sandwiches. Combine chopped nuts, mayonnaise, and celery in a chicken salad.

- Reserved Salmon Leftovers: For a quick and healthful dinner, flake the salmon and toss it with pasta, veggies, and a mild vinaigrette.

- Vegetables Leftover After Steaming: For a tasty stir-fry, sauté the vegetables with onions and garlic, add a source of protein, such as tofu or chickpeas, and serve over rice.

Reserved Roasted Potatoes: Chop the potatoes into small pieces, suitable for adding to omelets, frittatas, or breakfast hashes.

- Cooked Grains Leftovers: Make a grain salad by combining cooked grains such as brown rice or leftover quinoa with fresh veggies, herbs, and vinaigrette.

Dinner leftovers from the prior night provide a tasty, easy, and sustainable meal choice. You may optimize the benefits of leftovers and enjoy a range of delectable meals while minimizing food waste and saving money by paying attention to these pointers and investigating repurposing options.

CHAPTER FIVE

Dinnertime Dishes that Soothe and Satisfy

1. Baked salmon with roasted vegetables

A wholesome and filling dinner option, baked salmon with roasted veggies is a simple yet attractive dish that blends lean protein, vegetables high in fiber, and healthy fats. This dish's mild ingredients and cooking technique make it especially good for anyone with gastroesophageal reflux disease (GERD).

Benefits of Roasted Vegetables with Baked Salmon

- Slim Protein: Lean protein, such as salmon, is a great way to get the critical amino acids you need without consuming too much fat, which can worsen GERD symptoms. Additionally, it contains a lot of omega-3 fatty acids, which have anti-inflammatory qualities and may lower the chance of developing heart disease and other chronic illnesses.

- Vegetables High in Fibre: Adding fiber, vitamins, minerals, and antioxidants to a meal can be achieved by roasting a variety of vegetables. Fiber improves satiety, aids in digestion, and helps control blood sugar levels. The dish is more enticing because of the range of flavors and textures that roasted veggies bring to the table.

- Healthy Fats: The main fat used to roast veggies is olive oil, which is an excellent source of heart-healthy monounsaturated fats. It also gives the veggies more flavor and moisture.

- Slow Cooking Technique: Baking is a low-heat cooking technique that keeps the nutrients in the veggies and the salmon intact. Additionally, it stops the development of dangerous substances that may exacerbate GERD symptoms.

Choosing and Getting Ready for Salmon

For the most flavor and texture, go for fresh salmon filets. Choose salmon with the skin on because it shields the meat from heat and is simple to remove after baking.

- Time of Year: To taste, add more salt, pepper, and other herbs and spices to the salmon filets. You can enhance the flavor with paprika, garlic powder, or dried herbs like thyme or oregano.

- Heat of Cooking: For 12 to 15 minutes, or until the salmon is cooked through and flakes readily with a fork, bake it at a moderate 400°F (200°C).

Selecting and Preparing Vegetables

Choose a range of vibrant veggies to enhance the dish's taste and nutritional content. Select roasted veggies including onions, bell peppers, broccoli, carrots, and Brussels sprouts.

Cutting veggies: To guarantee uniform cooking, cut the veggies into pieces of the same size. Pieces that are smaller will roast faster.

- Time of Year: Mix the vegetables with more herbs or spices of your choice, olive oil, and salt and pepper.

- Heat of Roasting: Roast the vegetables for 20 to 30 minutes, or until they are soft and beginning to brown, at 400°F (200°C), the same temperature as the salmon.

Suggested Servings

For a full and well-balanced dinner, serve the baked salmon with roasted veggies and a side of healthful grains, like brown rice or quinoa. For added taste and nutrients, you can also sprinkle some balsamic vinegar or add a dollop of plain yogurt.

Guides for GERD-Friendly Meals Planning

- Steer clear of acidic ingredients: Tomatoes, citrus fruits, and pickles are examples of acidic foods to avoid since they can aggravate GERD symptoms.

- Reduce Fat: When roasting the vegetables, use a moderate amount of olive oil. To lessen the need for additional fat, you can also use a nonstick pan.

- Herbs and Spices for the Season: Herbs and spices such as oregano, basil, thyme, or a dash of black pepper can enhance the flavor of the salmon and veggies. Steer clear of strong spices or condiments that could aggravate the esophagus.

- Steer clear of creamy sauces: Simple condiments or sauces, like a balsamic reduction or a mild vinaigrette, are preferable than creamy sauces that could exacerbate GERD symptoms.

A tasty, nutrient-dense, and GERD-friendly dinner option is baked salmon with roasted veggies. You can eat this delectable food without jeopardizing your digestive comfort if you adhere to these instructions and tips.

2. Grilled chicken breast with quinoa and steamed asparagus

A healthy and filling dinner choice is grilled chicken breast with quinoa and steamed asparagus, which is a straightforward yet elegant recipe that blends lean protein, fiber-rich grains, and nutrient-dense veggies. Because of its delicate nature, this dish can be enjoyed by anyone with a variety of dietary requirements, including those who suffer from gastroesophageal reflux disease (GERD).

The advantages of combining grilled chicken breast with steamed asparagus and quinoa

- Limited Protein: Essential amino acids are provided by grilled chicken breast, but it doesn't include the extra fat that exacerbates GERD symptoms. Additionally, it is a good source of zinc, iron, and B vitamins.

- Quinoa Rich in Fibre: As a complete protein and high-fiber grain, quinoa facilitates digestion and encourages fullness. It is also a good source of iron, magnesium, and B vitamins, among other vitamins and minerals.

- High-Nutrient Asparagus: Asparagus offers fiber, antioxidants, vitamins, and minerals when steamed. This low-calorie vegetable gives the meal a subtle flavor and crunchy texture.

- Healthy Recipe Techniques: Steaming and grilling are low-heat cooking techniques that retain nutrients and stop the production of chemicals that can aggravate GERD symptoms.

Getting Ready to Grill a Chicken Breast

- Select Skinless Chicken Breast: For a reduced fat choice, go for skinless chicken breast.

- Marinate or Season: To enhance flavor, marinate the chicken breast in a blend of herbs, spices, and olive oil. Alternatively, just sprinkle salt and pepper on it.

- Sharpen to Excellence: Grill the chicken breast for four to five minutes on each side, or until it is cooked through and has some charring. Preheat the grill to medium-high heat.

Preparing Quinoa

- Clean and Prepare: To get rid of any bitterness, properly rinse the quinoa with water. Cook the quinoa as directed on the package, usually using a 1:2 quinoa to water ratio.

- Side notes and lingo: After cooking, use a fork to fluff the quinoa and add salt and pepper to taste.

Steamed Greens

- Trim and Wash: Remove the asparagus stalks' woody ends and give them a gentle wash.

- Steam Technique: Steam the asparagus for three to five minutes, or until it's crisp-tender, in a steamer basket set over boiling water.

Garnishing and Serving

- Mix and Present: Transfer the cooked quinoa, steaming asparagus, and grilled chicken breast to a platter.

- Garnish with Herbs: For extra taste and visual appeal, garnish the dish with fresh herbs like parsley, basil, or chives.

3. Turkey meatballs with whole-wheat pasta and marinara sauce

An easy way to make classic comfort food like turkey meatballs with whole-wheat spaghetti and marinara sauce better and more nutritious is to add some vegetables and other healthy ingredients. Lean ground turkey, whole-wheat pasta, and a homemade marinara sauce combine to make a dish that is easy on the stomach and high in fiber, protein, and other vital elements.

Turkey Meatballs with Marinara Sauce and Whole-Wheat Pasta Benefits

- Low Protein: Compared to beef or pig, ground turkey has less fat and still provides the necessary amino acids, without adding extra fat that can worsen the symptoms of GERD.

- Natural Pasta: Rich in fiber, whole-wheat pasta facilitates satiety, aids in digestion, and helps control blood sugar levels. Complex carbs are also included for long-term energy.

- Mericana Made at Home: Compared to store-bought sauces, homemade marinara sauce has fewer added sugars and preservatives and allows for greater ingredient control. The main ingredient in marinara sauce, tomatoes, are a good source of the antioxidant lycopene, which may have some health advantages.

- Programme of Balanced Macronutrients: With lean protein

from the turkey, fiber-rich whole-wheat pasta, and healthy fats from the olive oil used in the sauce, this dish offers a balanced macronutrient profile.

Making Meatballs with Turkey

- Select Turkey's Lean Ground Option: To reduce fat levels, choose ground turkey that is 90% or 93% lean.

- Tasty Fillings: To give the meatball mixture more taste and fiber, cut some veggies, like celery, carrots, and onions.

- Time of Year: Add salt, pepper, oregano, basil, and garlic powder to taste while seasoning the meatball mixture.

- Luminous Binding: To cut fat and cholesterol, use light binding components like oats, bread crumbs, or a flaxseed egg instead of heavy ones like eggs.

- Slow Cooking Technique: To reduce the amount of fat absorbed, bake or bake-fry the meatballs rather than deep-frying them.

Making Pasta with Whole Wheat

- Cook to Al Dente: Follow the instructions on the package to cook the whole-wheat pasta, trying to achieve an al dente texture that preserves firmness and nutrition.

- Remove and Throw: After cooking, rinse the pasta and toss it in a small amount of olive oil to add flavor and prevent sticking.

Creating Marinara Sauce at Home

- High-quality tomatoes: Use canned or fresh tomatoes to make the marinara sauce base. Nutrients and flavor are more vibrant in fresh tomatoes.

- Sauté veggies: To add taste and texture, sauté onions, garlic, and other desirable veggies, like bell peppers or zucchini, in olive oil.

To allow the flavors to blend, simmer the tomato mixture with herbs and spices like bay leaf, oregano, and basil along with salt and pepper.

- Adjust Consistency: You can thin out the sauce by cooking it longer to lower the liquid content or by adding water.

Garnishing and Serving

- Mix and Present: Transfer the cooked whole-wheat spaghetti, turkey meatballs, and marinara sauce into a serving dish.

- Picking Up Options: For extra taste and visual appeal, garnish the meal with fresh herbs like parsley, basil, or grated Parmesan cheese.

4. Veggie stir-fries with tofu or tempeh

Stir-fried vegetables are a flexible and simple-to-make dinner choice that can be tailored to fit different dietary requirements and palates. Using tofu or tempeh as the protein source gives this variant a pleasing texture and a nutritional boost, making it vegan-friendly and high in protein.

Veggie Stir-Fries with Tofu or Tempeh: Benefits

- Variety of veggies: Stir-fries are a great way to include a variety of veggies that are high in fiber, vitamins, and minerals.

- Protein Derived from Plants: Excellent plant-based protein sources that provide all the required amino acids without the cholesterol and saturated fat found in animal protein are tofu and tempeh.

- Low-Fat choice: Stir-fries are a low-fat supper choice that are easy on the stomach because they can be made with very little oil.

- Customization: Stir fries are a flexible and inclusive lunch option since they can be tailored to meet specific tastes and dietary requirements.

Selecting Veggies for Stir-Fries

Choose a range of vibrant veggies to enhance the stir-fry's taste and nutritional content. Choose stir-frying veggies like carrots, onions, bell peppers, broccoli florets, and mushrooms.

- Cutting veggies: To guarantee uniform cooking, cut the veggies into pieces of the same size. Pieces that are thinner will cook faster.

Getting Tempeh or Tofu Ready

The flavors of the other ingredients are absorbed by the neutral flavor of tofu and tempeh. Use these suggestions to improve their flavor and texture:

- Tofu: Tofu can be drained and pressed to eliminate extra moisture. Tofu can be crumbled or cubed to the desired texture. For added flavor, marinate the tofu in a mixture of sesame oil, ginger, garlic, and soy sauce.

- Tempeh: Slice or crumble tempeh into small pieces. For extra flavor, marinate the tempeh in a mixture of rice vinegar, soy sauce, tamari, ginger, and garlic.

Instant-Frying Method

For stir-fries, use a large skillet or hot wok to guarantee equal cooking and avoid sticking.

- Hume: In the wok or pan, warm up a tiny bit of vegetable or sesame oil over medium-high heat.

- Preparation Order: For a few minutes, start by stir-frying tougher veggies like broccoli florets or carrots. Add the softer veggies at the very end of cooking, like onions or bell peppers.

- Sauce Addition: In the final few minutes of cooking, add a stir-fry sauce or a straightforward concoction of soy sauce, rice vinegar, ginger, and garlic.

Suggested Servings

Serve the stir-fried vegetables with tofu or tempeh over cooked brown rice or quinoa to create a well-rounded and satisfying dinner. For an added crunch and nutritional boost, you may also mix in a small handful of chopped nuts or seeds.

Guides to a Tasty and Nutritious Stir-Fry

- Employ Fresh Substances: Choose seasonal, fresh veggies for maximum flavor and nutritional content.

- Sauces Variety: To add variation to your stir-fries, try experimenting with different sauces, such peanut sauce, teriyaki sauce, or a basic sauce made with soy sauce.

- Remember the salt: When adding sauces or seasonings, be aware of the amount of salt used. To taste, adjust the salt content.

Stir-fried vegetables with tempeh or tofu provide a tasty, plant-based dinner option. You can make tasty stir-fries that are full of plant-based protein, healthy fats, and vegetables by using these suggestions and principles.

5. Lentil soup with whole-grain bread

For ages, lentil soup has been a staple in many cultures due to its hardiness and flavor. It is a great option for a filling and healthful lunch because it is full of protein, fiber, and other important elements. Together with whole-grain bread, this combination makes for a satisfying and well-balanced lunch choice.

Advantages of Whole-Grain Bread with Lentil Soup

- High Protein Content: Plant-based protein sources like lentils are a great way to get the essential amino acids needed for muscle growth and repair.

- High Fiber Content: A great source of fiber that facilitates satiety, aids in digestion, and helps control blood sugar levels is lentils.

- High in Nutrients: Iron, potassium, and B vitamins are among the many vitamins and minerals that are abundant in lentils.

- Grain Bread: Whole: In addition to providing more fiber, whole-grain bread also contains vitamins, minerals, and complex carbs for long-lasting energy.

- Solace Meal: A warm and soothing dish like lentil soup is ideal for a cozy dinner on a chilly day.

Making Soup with Lentils

Because it's so easy to make, lentil soup is a great option for weeknight dinners or informal weekend gatherings.

- Seeds: To get a range of tastes and textures, combine green, red, and yellow lentils. Rinse the lentils well to make sure all the debris is gone.

- Vegetables: Choose a range of vibrant veggies to infuse the soup with taste and nutrients. Carrots, celery, onions, and tomatoes are typical options.

- Time of Year: Add herbs and spices to taste, such as bay leaf, thyme, oregano, and salt and pepper to the soup.

- Preparation Technique: Once the lentils are soft, simmer them with the vegetables in vegetable broth. You can thin down the soup by adding extra broth or cooking it longer to lessen the amount of liquid.

To Serve: Whole-Grain Bread

Combine your lentil soup with whole-grain bread to create a well-rounded and satisfying dinner.

- Bread Selection: Choose whole grain breads with low levels of processed carbs and high levels of fiber. To be sure the bread is mostly produced with whole-wheat flour, look for labels that say "whole-wheat" or "100% whole-wheat."

- Options for Serving: Cut the whole-grain bread into slices and present it with the lentil soup, ready to be dipped or spread with hummus or light butter.

- Additional Garnishes: Add chopped fresh herbs, such as parsley or dill, to the soup to improve its flavor and presentation.

Recipe for a Tasty and Nutritious Lentil Soup

- Sauté veggies: To improve the flavor and texture of the veggies, sauté them in a tiny bit of olive oil before adding them to the soup.

- Seasoning Adjustments: Taste the soup as it cooks and make any necessary adjustments to the seasoning.

- Think About Adding More Protein: For a more protein-rich dinner, feel free to add extra protein sources to the soup, such as cooked lean chicken or tofu.

Whole-grain bread paired with lentil soup makes a satisfying, wholesome, and simple supper alternative. You may make a tasty and filling dinner that is full of fiber, protein, and other important nutrients by using these suggestions and principles.

CHAPTER SIX

Sample Meal Plans for a GERD-Friendly Lifestyle

1. A week-long meal plan incorporating breakfast, lunch, dinner, and snacks

Day 1

Lunch:

- Berries and nuts with muesli: This traditional meal is loaded with protein and fiber to keep you going all morning. As directed on the package, prepare the muesli, then garnish with chopped nuts and a few fresh or frozen berries for some crunch and beneficial fats.

Snack:

- Fruit and granola with Greek yogurt: Granola and fruit offer healthy carbohydrates and fiber, while Greek yogurt is a terrific source of protein. Add granola for sweetness and texture, then top plain Greek yogurt with a selection of fresh or frozen fruits.

Lunch:

- Grilled chicken or tofu salad: This nutrient-dense salad is a light and refreshing lunch choice. For an added protein boost, mix grilled chicken or tofu with chopped veggies and mixed greens. Use a lemon-tahini sauce or a light vinaigrette to dress the salad.

Supper:

- Roasted veggies and baked salmon: This is a tasty and nutritious option for dinner. Roast a variety of veggies, including Brussels sprouts, broccoli, and carrots, to go with the baked salmon filets.

Day 2

Lunch:

- Avocado and whole-wheat bread with scrambled eggs: This is a simple, quick meal that is rich in healthy fats and protein. Serve scrambled eggs with sliced avocado on whole-wheat bread, topped with your preferred vegetables.

Snack:

- Slices of apple with almond butter: Almond butter offers protein and excellent lipids, and apple slices are a wonderful source of antioxidants and fiber. For a filling snack, combine apple slices with a tablespoon of almond butter.

Lunch:

Whole-grain bread and lentil soup: A filling and healthy lunch choice that is high in protein and fiber is lentil soup. For an additional boost of fiber and carbohydrates, serve it with a side of whole-grain bread.

Supper:

- Marinara sauce and whole-wheat pasta paired with turkey meatballs: Made with healthier ingredients, this is a family-friendly favorite. Serve turkey meatballs with homemade marinara sauce over whole-wheat spaghetti, baked or baked-fried.

Day 3

Lunch:

- Fruit, yogurt, and spinach smoothie: A healthy and easy way to start the day is with this smoothie. Smoothie: Blend spinach, yogurt, and your favorite fruit for a high-fiber, high-protein smoothie.

Snack:

- Hummus on carrots: Carrots are high in fiber and minerals, and hummus is high in protein and beneficial fats. For a filling snack, try carrot sticks with a side of hummus.

Lunch:

Veggie wrap with tofu or grilled chicken: This wrap makes a tasty and convenient lunch choice. For a high-protein lunch, top grilled chicken or tofu with chopped vegetables and mixed greens within a whole-wheat tortilla.

Supper:

- Brown rice and tofu or tempeh stir-fried: A quick and simple dinner that's high in protein and vegetables is this stir-fry. Stir-fry a range of veggies with tempeh or tofu, including bell peppers, carrots, and broccoli. For a full supper, serve the stir-fry over brown rice.

Day 4

Lunch:

- Chia seeds and fruit overnight oats: For a quick and healthful breakfast, try overnight oats. Put your favorite fruit, yogurt, chia seeds, milk, and rolled oats in a jar, then chill overnight. The flavors will seep into the oats, resulting in a quick and simple breakfast that can be eaten on the go.

Snack:

- Nut and seed trail mix with dried fruit: Trail mix is a healthy, portable snack that is high in fiber, protein, and good fats. To make your own trail mix, mix nuts, seeds, and dried fruit together.

Lunch:

- Whole-grain crackers paired with black bean soup: A satisfying and tasty lunch option that is high in fiber and protein is black bean soup. For an additional boost of fiber and carbohydrates, serve it alongside whole-grain crackers.

Supper:

- Grilled chicken breast paired with roasted veggies and quinoa: This meal option is balanced and healthful. Alongside grilled chicken breasts that are cooked through, roast a variety of vegetables, including bell peppers, zucchini, and asparagus. For a full dinner, serve the chicken and veggies over quinoa.

Day 5

Lunch:

- Fruit and whole-wheat pancakes with eggs: This breakfast is full, well-balanced, and packed with fiber and protein. Serve your preferred vegetables-topped scrambled eggs alongside whole-wheat pancakes that have been dusted with frozen or fresh fruit.

Snack:

- Sprouts and avocado on rice cakes: The low-fat rice cakes.

Day 6

Lunch:

- Whole-wheat tortilla, eggs, black beans, and salsa in a breakfast burrito:** This breakfast burrito is a tasty, portable choice that's high in fiber and protein. Top a whole-wheat tortilla with your preferred toppings, salsa, black beans, and scrambled eggs.

Snack:

- Hummus-topped veggie sticks:** Carrots, celery, and cucumber sticks are excellent sources of vitamins and fiber; hummus, on the other hand, offers protein and healthful fats. For a filling snack, serve veggie sticks with a side of hummus.

Lunch:

- Whole-grain bread with tofu salad sandwich: This sandwich is a flavorful plant-based protein alternative. Combine diced veggies, mashed avocado, crumbled tofu, and a mild vinaigrette. Spread the mixture of tofu over whole-grain bread for a filling and healthy meal.

Supper:

- Salmon baked with Brussels sprouts and roasted sweet potatoes:** This is a tasty and nutritious option for dinner. Toss in some sweet potatoes and Brussels sprouts and bake the salmon filets until done.

Day 7

Lunch:

- Nuts and fruit with whole-wheat waffles: Waffles made from whole wheat are a terrific way to start the day with complex carbohydrates and fiber, and they're healthier than regular waffles. For extra taste and nutrition, top your waffles with frozen or fresh fruit and a sprinkling of almonds.

Snack:

- Pearl and granola with cottage cheese: Protein-rich cottage cheese is a fantastic combination with fiber-rich oats and nutritious carbs from pineapple. For a filling and healthy snack, mix diced pineapple with cottage cheese and top with oats.

Lunch:

- Remaining lentil soup accompanied by a side salad: A quick and simple lunch option that is high in protein and fiber is leftover lentil soup. For additional fiber and vegetables, serve it with a side salad.

Supper:

- Grilled chicken paired with quinoa and roasted veggies: This meal option is balanced and healthful. Roast drumsticks or thighs of chicken until they are cooked through, and roast potatoes, carrots, and onions to go with them. For a full dinner, serve the chicken and veggies over quinoa.

Snacks:

- Fresh fruit: For a wholesome and revitalizing snack, always have a range of fresh fruit on hand. Oranges, bananas, berries, and apples are all excellent choices.

- Vegetables: For a nutritious and crisp snack, always have a range of vegetables on hand. Bell peppers, cucumbers, celery, and carrots are all healthy choices.

- Nuts and seeds: Rich in fiber, protein, and beneficial fats, nuts and seeds are a great food. Good choices include almonds, walnuts, peanuts, sunflower seeds, and pumpkin seeds.

- Yogurt: Rich in calcium and protein, yogurt is a great food. For a filling snack, try plain yogurt with your preferred fruit or topped with granola.

This meal plan is merely an example; you can modify it to your own plan.

2. Tips for planning and preparing meals ahead of time

Planning

1. Assess your schedule: Look at your forthcoming week and note the days when you'll be short on time for cooking before you begin meal planning. This will assist you in prioritizing the meals that need to be prepared in advance.

2. Take into account your preferences: Pick meals that are convenient to keep and reheat for you and your family. Make sure to account for any dietary requirements or limits you may have.

3. Make a variety plan: Avoid falling into a routine where you eat the same thing every day. To guarantee you're getting a range of nutrients and to keep things interesting, switch up your meals.

4. Make a list of things to buy: Make a shopping list with all the ingredients you'll need once you've decided on your

menu. You'll save money and time at the grocery shop by doing this.

Readiness

1. Cook in bulk: Making meals in bulk is a fantastic method to save down on preparation time. Once a grain, protein, or vegetable is cooked in bulk, it can be used for several meals during the week.

2. Prepare and chop vegetables: Prepare and chop veggies in advance so they're ready to use when you're ready to cook. Cooking will become considerably simpler and faster as a result.

3. Saute once, consume twice: Make twice as much food as needed and freeze half for later. When you're pressed for time, this is a terrific way to have simple, quick meals on hand.

4. Make sensible use of leftovers: Avoid wasting leftovers. Use them to create new dishes or store them for the next day's lunch.

Reserve

1. Use airtight containers: To keep food fresher for longer and avoid spoiling, store it in airtight containers.

2. Label and date food: Make sure you label and date every food item so you can identify what it is and when it was prepared.

3. Freeze correctly: To avoid freezer burn, freeze food in freezer bags or sealed containers.

You can simply plan and prepare meals in advance by using these suggestions, which will help you save time and reduce stress in the kitchen.

3. Strategies for eating out and ordering takeout without triggering GERD symptoms

Pick the Correct Restaurant

- Select GERD-friendly food options: Give preference to eateries that feature healthful grains, steamed or roasted veggies, and lean protein sources in their menus. Seek out establishments that specialize in vegetarian, Asian, or Mediterranean food.

- Avoid trigger foods: As fried foods, creamy sauces, rich sweets, and spicy dishes are major causes of GERD symptoms, avoid dining at establishments that prominently emphasize them.

Make Well-Informed Menu Selections

- Steamed or grill-cooked protein: Lean protein options like chicken, fish, or tofu that are grilled or steamed are preferable to those that are fried or breaded.

- Veggie-heavy dishes: Pick meals that are heavy on the veggies, particularly those that are roasted or steam-cooked. Steer clear of buttery recipes and thick cream sauces.

- Complete grain selections: For optimal fiber and vitamin content, use whole-grain sides such as brown rice, quinoa, or whole-wheat bread.

- Dark overlays: Instead of creamy or thick sauces on salads, ask for light dressings or vinaigrettes.

- Reduce the number of acidic elements in the dish: Steer clear of recipes that contain a lot of tomatoes, citrus fruits, or pickles as they might make GERD symptoms worse.

Keep in Touch with Your Server.

- Inform about GERD: Let your server know that you have GERD and enquire about the ingredients and cooking techniques used in particular meals.

- Make changes request: Never be afraid to ask for dish adjustments, such as taking out sauces, keeping cheese, or grilling rather than frying.

- Request choices without gluten: Ask about gluten-free options or whether it's possible to prepare recipes using gluten-free substitutes if you have a gluten sensitivity.

Purchasing Takeout Sensibly

- Examine online menus: Examine internet menus for restaurants in advance to make well-informed decisions and steer clear of possible triggers.

- Indicate your preferences: Make sure to specify any dietary restrictions or preferences when placing a takeaway order in order to reduce the risk of GERD symptoms.

- Select healthful sides: Choose salads with light dressings, whole-grain alternatives, or steamed veggies as light and healthful sides.

- Avoid late-night takeaway:** Avoid ordering takeaway right before bed since it can exacerbate symptoms of GERD.

- Warn to reheat: Reheating takeaway should be done carefully; using too much heat or overcooking can change the flavors and nutritional value.

You may enjoy eating out and ordering takeaway without aggravating your GERD symptoms by using these tips. Always pay attention to what your body tells you, and select foods that suit your dietary requirements and preferences.

CHAPTER SIX

Lifestyle Habits that Complement a GERD-Friendly Diet

1. Maintaining a healthy weight

Sustaining a healthy weight lowers the chance of developing a number of chronic diseases and is essential for general wellbeing. It entails striking a balance between the number of calories consumed and expended in order to reach a weight that is suitable for your height, age, and sex. The following are some practical methods for keeping a healthy weight:

1. Give nutrient-dense foods priority: Make a point of eating nutrient-dense

whole foods like fruits, vegetables, whole grains, and lean protein sources. Avoid processed and packaged foods. These foods sustain general health by providing vital vitamins, minerals, and fiber to keep you full and energized.

2. Limit Processed meals: Reduce the amount of sugar-filled beverages, processed meals, and harmful fats that you consume. These foods can lead to weight gain and health problems because they are frequently low in nutrients and high in calories.

3. Employ Portion Control Techniques: Pay attention to portion proportions to prevent overindulging. To determine the right portions, use measuring cups or a food scale, and pay attention to your body's signals of hunger and fullness.

4. Include Frequent Physical Activity: Exercise on a regular basis to increase

your muscle mass and burn calories. Try to get in at least 150 minutes a week of moderate-to-intense aerobic activity or 75 minutes a week of strenuous aerobic activity. Incorporate strength training activities to improve metabolism and muscular tone.

5. Monitor Your Weight: Weigh yourself on a regular basis to keep tabs on your weight and see any patterns. For long-term weight loss or maintenance, set reasonable weight goals and gradually adjust your food and exercise routine.

6. Seek Professional Guidance: For individualized guidance on maintaining a healthy weight and eating well, speak with a licensed dietitian or nutritionist. They can assist you in designing a customized strategy that fits your unique requirements and preferences.

7. Talk About the Basis Conditions: Work with your healthcare practitioner to properly manage any underlying medical disorders, such as hypothyroidism or polycystic ovarian syndrome (PCOS), that may impact your ability to manage your weight.

8. Make Sleep a Priority: Try to get 7-8 hours of good sleep every night. Getting enough sleep aids in the regulation of hormones that govern metabolism and appetite, which supports weight control.

9. Effective Stress Management: Prolonged stress might impede attempts to lose weight and contribute to weight gain. Look for stress-reduction techniques that are beneficial, including yoga, meditation, or outdoor activities.

10. Make Sustainable Lifestyle Changes: Rather than concentrating on band-aid solutions, make sustainable

lifestyle changes. For long-term success, gradually introduce and sustain healthy habits into your daily routine.

Recall that keeping a healthy weight is a process rather than a goal. As you strive towards your objectives, treat yourself with kindness, patience, and consistency. Along the process, acknowledge your accomplishments and ask for help when you need it.

2. Managing stress levels

Stress is a normal reaction to demanding or difficult circumstances. It can show up physically, emotionally, or behaviorally and be brought on by a variety of circumstances, both good and bad. A certain amount of stress can be good for us, but too much or chronic stress can be bad for our health and wellbeing.

Determining the Stressors

Finding out what causes your stress response is the first step towards controlling stress. These pressures might be internal, like perfectionism, anxiety, or self-criticism, or external, such as marital problems, work deadlines, or money worries.

Practical Stress Reduction Techniques

1. Daily Activity: Being physically active is a great way to decompress. On most days of the week, work out for at least 30 minutes at a moderate to high level. Endorphins are released during exercise and are known to improve mood and reduce stress.

2. Meditation and Mindfulness: Deep breathing exercises and other mindfulness techniques can help reduce stress hormones, quiet the mind, and foster inner peace. Set aside some time every day to clear your head and concentrate on the here and now.

3. Responsible Sleep: Getting enough sleep is crucial for managing stress. Try to get between seven and eight hours of good sleep per night to give your body time to recuperate. Create a calming nighttime routine and stick to a regular sleep schedule.

4. Relaxation Techniques: Practice gradual muscle relaxation, yoga, or tai chi as relaxation techniques. These techniques aid in promoting mental calm and releasing physical tension.

5. Organization and Time Management: Good time management keeps you from

feeling overburdened, which lowers stress. Prioritize your work, make a plan for the day, and don't put things off. Divide complex tasks into smaller, more doable segments.

6. Social Linkage: Strong social ties ease stress and offer assistance. Develop your bonds with loved ones, family, and friends. Take part in activities that promote belonging and social connection.

7. Optimal Nutrition: A balanced diet can aid in stress management and promote general well being. Eat a lot of whole grains, fruits, and veggies. Restrict processed foods, sugar-filled beverages, and high caffeine intake.

8. Ask for Expert Assistance: If stress is having a negative effect on your life, you should think about getting professional treatment. A therapist can offer direction

and encouragement for stress management and coping strategy development.

Extra Advice on Handling Stress:

- Determine the specific stressors that affect your own stress management and create plans to either avoid or effectively manage them.

- Avoid self-criticism and cultivate self-compassion. Recognise your tension, but try not to focus on it.

- Take part in enjoyable and relaxing activities. Allocate time for interests, hobbies, and recreational pursuits.

- Don't take on more than you can handle and instead set reasonable expectations for yourself.

- Acquire the ability to decline more obligations when it becomes necessary to put your health first.

- When assistance is required, ask friends, relatives, or a support group for it.

Recall that managing stress is a continuous endeavor. Try out several methods and see which one suits you the best. Prioritize your well-being, have patience with yourself, and make small, steady improvements.

3. Quitting smoking

One of the best things you can do for your health is to stop smoking. There are a lot of short- and long-term advantages associated with stopping smoking.

Quick Advantages:

- Better respiratory and lung function, Lower risk of heart attack and stroke, Enhanced taste and smell perception, Lower chance of cancer

Enduring Advantages:

- Extended life expectancy, Decreased chance of acquiring chronic illnesses like diabetes, heart disease, stroke, and lung cancer, Better general health and wellbeing

Getting Ready to Give Up Smoking

Although giving up smoking is difficult, it is achievable with the correct planning and assistance. The following actions can help you become ready to stop:

1. Set a quit date: Write down a date that works for you, preferably in the near future. This will allow you enough time to emotionally and psychologically get ready to stop.

2. Determine your triggers: What circumstances or feelings usually make you want to light up? You can create plans to prevent or control your triggers if you are aware of them.

3. Speak with your physician: Inform your physician of your intentions to stop smoking. In addition to offering guidance and support, they could recommend medicine to aid in your quitting.

4. Acquire support Inform your loved ones about your intention to resign. They can support you and help you remain on course.

5. Select a method of quitting: There are numerous approaches to stop smoking, including nicotine replacement therapy (NRT), counseling, and cold turkey. Select the approach you believe will be most effective for you.

Smoking Cessation Techniques

After you're ready, try these tips to help you stop smoking:

1. Eliminate temptation: Take out all ashtrays and smokes from your vehicle, house, and place of employment.

2. Avoid triggers: Recognise the things that make you want to smoke and try to stay away from them. Have a strategy for handling a trigger if you are unable to avoid it.

3. Find healthy alternatives: Instead of smoking, switch to healthy pursuits like

walking, working out, or quality time with loved ones.

4. Have patience: It takes time and effort to stop smoking. Don't give up if you make a mistake. Simply get back up and go again.

5. Seek support: When you're in need, talk to your physician, a counselor, or other members of the support group.

Remind yourself that giving up smoking is one of the most difficult but gratifying things you will ever do. With the correct planning, encouragement, and techniques, you can permanently stop smoking and get the health benefits for years to come.

Conclusion

The persistent reflux of stomach contents into the esophagus is the hallmark of gastroesophageal reflux disease (GERD), a common digestive ailment. The esophagus lining may become irritated by this reflux of acid, leading to a variety of painful symptoms, such as:

- Heartburn: a scorching feeling that frequently travels to the throat

- Recapitulation: The mouthfeel of gastric acid, which is sour or bitter

- Dysphagia, or difficulty swallowing

- Heart ache

- Persistent cough

- Sibilant Voice

GERD Contributing Factors

The lower esophageal sphincter (LES), a muscle valve that keeps stomach contents from draining back into the esophagus, is the main cause of GERD. Acid reflux from the stomach can irritate and inflame the esophagus when the LES weakens or relaxes improperly.

GERD can be caused by various reasons, including as:

- Hiatal hernia: A disorder that weakens the LES when the upper portion of the stomach pushes through the diaphragm, the muscle that divides the chest from the abdomen.

- Fatality: Being overweight can raise the pressure inside the abdomen, which pushes the stomach up and weakens the LES.

- Growth: Pregnancy-related hormonal changes may loosen the LES and raise the risk of GERD.

- Specific drugs: Drugs that relax the LES, such as beta-blockers and muscle relaxants, can exacerbate GERD symptoms.

- Cigarette Use: Smoking increases the risk of reflux by irritating the esophagus and weakening the LES.

Dietary Adjustments and Lifestyle Modifications for the Management of GERD

Even though GERD can be a chronic ailment, there are ways to greatly manage symptoms and enhance overall health with food and lifestyle adjustments. Here are a few crucial suggestions:

- Avoid trigger foods: Recognise and steer clear of foods that aggravate GERD symptoms, such as heartburn. Chocolate, citrus fruits, tomatoes, chocolate, spicy or fatty foods, and caffeine are common triggers.

- Keep your weight in check: Being overweight might exacerbate the symptoms of GERD by putting more strain on the stomach. Maintain a healthy weight range by eating a well-balanced diet and getting frequent exercise.

- Consume smaller, more regular meals: Large meals can cause the stomach to become overloaded and raise the chance of reflux. To encourage healthy digestion, choose to eat smaller, more frequent meals throughout the day.

- Avoid eating late at night: Give your stomach enough time to process meals before going to sleep. If you want to lessen the chance of reflux at night, avoid eating for three to four hours after lying down.

- Raise the head of your bed: To stop stomach acid from refluxing back into the esophagus while you sleep, raise the head of your bed by 6 to 8 inches.

- Thoroughly chew food: Chewing food breaks it down into tiny bits, which facilitates stomach digestion and lowers the chance of reflux.

- Refrain from smoking: Smoking can exacerbate the symptoms of GERD by weakening the LES and irritating the lining of the stomach. Giving up smoking might greatly enhance GERD treatment.

GERD Treatment Medication

Medication may be recommended in addition to dietary and lifestyle changes to control GERD symptoms and avoid problems. Typical drugs consist of:

- Acidifiers: Antacids, such as Tums and Mylanta, neutralize stomach acid and offer immediate relief from the symptoms of heartburn.

- H2 blockers: H2 blockers, including Pepcid and Zantac, lessen the formation of stomach acid and provide longer-lasting relief.

- Inhibitors of proton pump action (PPIs): The most effective drugs for lowering acid production are proton pump inhibitors (PPIs), like Nexium and Prilosec, which can relieve severe GERD over time.

Looking for Expert Advice on GERD

For an accurate diagnosis and course of therapy, it is imperative that you speak with a healthcare provider if you are exhibiting symptoms of GERD. Barrett's esophagus, esophageal ulcers, and an increased risk of esophageal cancer are among the consequences that can be avoided with early intervention and management.

Recall that, with the appropriate care, GERD is a treatable illness. You can effectively control symptoms, enhance your quality of life, and avoid long-term consequences by implementing dietary adjustments, lifestyle changes, and medication when needed.

www.ingramcontent.com/pod-product-compliance
Lightning Source LLC
Chambersburg PA
CBHW070932260726
48661CB00003B/947